Bad Eye

A journey of eye surgery and visual impairment

Susan Fisher

Disclaimer: I am not a doctor and the opinions and thoughts shared in this personal narrative describe my own journey of eye surgery and visual impairment. If you feel you have a vision issue or other health concern, please visit your eye doctor or health professional for advice, diagnosis, and treatment.

Table of Contents

Chapter One:
Begin at the Beginning

How do you tell a story about losing your eyesight? I guess the easiest way is to begin at the beginning. But that's hard to do when you don't know when or where the beginning was. Did it happen when I stepped inside after shoveling snow? It was an early and wet snowfall. I didn't realize the soles of both shoes were caked with snow. I stepped into the house onto an area rug and walked across the room. It was only when I stepped onto the hardwood floor on the other side that I felt my feet flying out from under me. I lurched forward and it seemed like time was suspended as I tried to right myself. I remember thinking, "Oh my gosh, I'm not going to right myself, I'm going to fall," which I think is what every adult thinks when they realize they are going down. I hit the floor face down but mostly caught myself with my hands and arms. I stayed there for a few minutes. I moved each arm and then my legs to make sure nothing was broken. I felt my face and didn't feel any pain, so I got up. I was fine.

Another possibility I considered was when I helped my man move some really heavy furniture. I know "my man" sounds archaic and implies ownership, but when you are older and not married, all of the other terms don't seem to fit and seem odd. Partner sounds ambiguous. Boyfriend sounds like you are still in high school. Significant other sounds odd. Manfriend sounds made up, like merman (as in *Zoolander*.) So usually, I just say "my man." Anyway, we moved some really heavy furniture one weekend. Another thing you should know is that this relationship is long distance, even though it didn't start that way. For some, long distance is the wrong distance, but it works for us, so we stay together. The day after moving the furniture, I was in Chicago on my way back home. I was in Union Station and happened to look down at my hands. They looked bluish to me. Was I seeing things? No, it wasn't the fluorescent lighting in the Great Hall, the palms of my hands were actually bruised. If I strained myself that hard moving furniture maybe I had also strained the retina in my right eye.

In hindsight, other possibilities could have been to blame. All I knew was that I started to see something, but I didn't know what it was, in my right eye. I wasn't alarmed when I saw it, I just didn't know what it was. It was like a little dark flag or pennant wavering around at the top of my vision. "Ugh!" When I read descriptions now of the HUGE red flags that tell you your retina is detaching, the descriptions always mention a curtain or a shadow. Now it seems so obvious that I was seeing exactly that.

I already had my annual eye appointment scheduled for the next week. Since I wasn't concerned about the little wiggly thing in my vision, I didn't call to see my optometrist sooner. Cue some ominous music here, because apparently when you have a detached retina, minutes and hours can make the difference in your visual outcome.

At the eye doctor's, there was a new piece of equipment. It provided internal imaging, but it wasn't covered by my insurance and would cost an extra $10 out of pocket. I opted to include it in the exam. My eye doctor was pleasant as always. She conducted the exam as usual and I told her I was seeing something in my right eye. She said maybe it was just too much computer time at work. I'm the public relations specialist for the public library system in my town. It surprises people sometimes that there is a PR position at the library system in a smallish community, but we have four branches, provide an abundance of excellent programming, and seek out grants on the local, state, and national levels. So I am always busy. There are lots of words (and pictures and videos) to communicate to the public on lots of levels. Writing to a sixth-grade reader is the norm for newspaper press releases, while applying for grants, especially technical and computer equipment grants, requires a higher level of writing.

The eye doctor told me I should take more breaks while working and to make sure I spent more time looking away from the computer screen. She thought the problem would resolve itself. By this time, the results from the new eye imaging equipment popped up on her computer. She leaned into the screen and looked concerned. "What are you doing when you leave here?" she asked. I told her I was going to treat myself to something at the bakery across the street on my way to work. "There's been a change in plans," she said. "I don't see this often, but I think you may have a detached retina. We need to get you to a specialist immediately." She got on the phone to the front receptionist and asked her to find out which retina specialists might be open for an immediate appointment. While we waited, she asked me if anything had happened recently. A blow to the head? A car accident? A sports injury? I was too panicked to think back to some of the things that could have been the cause. She said any intense strain could have caused it, even straining hard while using the bathroom. That comment stays with me to this day and causes concern anytime I may feel constipated.

The eye doctor said there were two retina specialists in town and lucky for me one would see me immediately. I left the office in a daze and called work to let them know I wouldn't be in right away and I would keep them posted. Next, I called my oldest sister. She is an eye doctor in Seattle. I wanted her input right away. She was probably on her way to work, given our three-hour time difference, and didn't answer.

I walked into the retina specialist's office and was immediately underwhelmed. It was part of a strip mall kind of office development and the interior was not impressive. Another sister (not the eye doctor) owns a laser spa, and I had helped her consider the interiors and renovations at leased spaces. This office space looked a bit tired around the edges, with worn carpet and dark paneling. The specialist himself seemed friendly enough. He examined both eyes, obviously with more attention to the right eye. He used a piece of equipment for imagery. As we waited for the results, he said based on his visual exam, he wasn't sure that it would be a detached retina but rather retinoschisis. He pronounced the end of the word "schisis" in a way that sounded like a bad impression of someone speaking German. I had a really bad feeling, and I wanted to be anywhere other than where I was.

When he came back in with the results of the imaging, the retinoschisis idea was thrown out and he declared that I did, in fact, have a detached retina and it needed surgery. Immediately. He left the room to consult his surgery schedule. My phone rang. It was my sister, the eye doctor. I told her what was happening and told her some of the

8

technical terms he had used to describe it. I told her surgery and scleral buckle were mentioned. She said given the diagnosis, this sounded like the needed course of action. The retina specialist came back to the room and handed me a clipboard with a stack of forms that I needed to sign for a surgery that would take place the next morning. I was in shock as I signed the forms and drove to the local hospital.

The pre-op tests were completed. Weight, height, blood pressure, etc. It was a blur. I returned home and called work and my mom. I would need a ride to and from surgery. I needed to be off work for 30 days, which sounded like a lifetime. It was hard to comprehend. Just that morning, I thought I would be out of the office for a few hours for a checkup and now my life was going to be turned upside down for 30 days. It seemed insurmountable. In hindsight, 30 days would have been a walk in the park.

Later that afternoon, my sister, the laser spa owner, called. "Don't do it," she said. "Don't have surgery with this local doctor. Go get a second opinion." See, in addition to her spa, she also does lasering one day a week at an eye center in Indianapolis. She said the surgeons at the center were often consulted after patients were unhappy with their visual outcomes following surgeries at local, smaller hospitals. I was already on edge and growing anxious about the scheduled surgery. Everything was happening so fast and I just wanted it to be over. I told her I had talked to a friend whose husband, a construction company owner, had a sudden retinal detachment. The surgeon I was working with had repaired it quickly and adeptly. Her husband couldn't even tell which eye had been affected. The outcome was excellent. I told my sister I was sticking with the surgeon I had been referred to.

Later, the receptionist at the large eye institute called. She said that my sister had begged her to convince me that I was making a mistake to go through with the surgery. Even later still, my eye doctor sister called and joined in the chorus that I should see someone else. I told her I knew about others with good outcomes and I had already gone through all of the pre-op tests and I just wanted this to be over as quickly as possible. I tossed and turned all night.

My mom took me to the local hospital early the next morning. I hadn't eaten or had anything to drink since midnight the night before. This is pretty standard for surgery. If you cough or choke during the surgery, they don't want anything in your stomach to end up in your lungs. When they called my name, my mom and I both approached the patient entrance door. "Don't worry Susan, everything will be just fine," said the nurse as she took my mom's arm in a gentle and caring manner. "Thanks," I said, "but I'm Susan and that nice lady is my mom." The nurse pulled her arm back in surprise. This became a familiar scenario over the next few years. People automatically assumed the younger person was there to assist the older person.

As I lay on the gurney before being wheeled into the operating room, I started to cry. One of the surgical nurses tried to comfort me. I told her that everyone I know and love had told me to cancel the surgery and to get a second opinion at a specialty eye clinic. To her credit, she said, "Honey, if you don't feel good about this, say so right now. You can change your mind." I told her no, that I was sure I was doing the right thing and, in my mind, having surgery sooner meant this would all be over sooner.

I would be completely under for the surgery, so crying in the hallway is about all I remember. The surgery was outpatient, so within a few hours I was on my way home with my mom at the wheel. We stopped at a local drugstore with the multiple prescriptions for the needed eye drops. This is when I was introduced to the eye drop world and the lingo of pink tops, yellow tops, and red tops. It's a secret language I never knew about, but something all those in the world of eye surgery know and understand. The drop schedule was different for each color of top and function of the drop. I was back home with the right eye severely patched and taped and with a special foam tray/pillow thingie that would help me to position as needed to help the recovery process. I immediately went to bed, so I could follow the strict rules for positioning. This means laying in the position instructed by your doctor and your position depends on where the retinal tear was. For me, that meant laying on my left side. I was allowed to get up for 10 minutes of each hour. That gave me enough time to use the eye drops as needed, let my dog out, use the bathroom, and maybe grab something to eat. No one tells you how hard it is to position for several days. By the end of day two, my left shoulder, elbow, knee, hip, and ankle felt like they were on fire. When I looked online for ideas to make the positioning more tolerable, there wasn't a whole lot of advice. One site said to remember to keep your head down and your spirits up! I suspected this bon mot wasn't created by someone who was actually positioning, and when advised to someone who was positioning, created a strong desire in the patient to punch whoever was offering it as cheery encouragement.

The first morning after the surgery, I took a picture of my face. I still had the eye patch on and the swelling of my entire face was not pretty. I sent it to my man. "Wow," he texted back, "so this was like surgery, surgery, not some laser thing?" It was real alright. "And why do your lips look so big?" he asked. "Wait, what?" I sent the picture to my sister with the laser spa. She texted back, "Your face looks like a mess but your lips look awesome and big!" I assured everyone that I was not offered lip fillers or injections as part of the eye surgery but wondered if maybe the surgeon had stood on my face to almost practically pop my eye out of its socket so he could stitch the scleral buckle onto the back of it. The buckle is supposed to squeeze the eye and help keep the retina in place.

At some point, I should share that I am one of the most squeamish people I know. Yes, I was able to give birth to two wonderful daughters, but I have always been squeamish about anything involving blood or anything medical. In a required biology course in college, I was in a huge lecture hall where the professor was showing slides that looked kind of like those transparent overlays of human organs. I felt the room spin and had to put my head between my knees to keep from passing out. Growing up, we had a set of the World Book Encyclopedias that had similar transparencies. I knew exactly where those pages were and always turned away and flipped past them really quickly so I wouldn't accidentally see them.

So for me to deal with a messy, gooey looking eye was torture. By the third day after the surgery, I was able to leave the patch off and for the first time I stood at my bathroom mirror and really looked at it. What a mess! The eye literally looked like hamburger. I gently pulled on my eyelid to see even more of the eyeball. But the eyeball was still so swollen and misshapen that I couldn't even see a curve that meant the blob was still shaped like an eyeball. Worse still, as I leaned in closer, I noticed a little black something sticking out from the surface of the eyeball. "What the heck? Is that a piece of fuzz or something from my sweatshirt?" I touched it very carefully with my finger. "Oh my gosh!" It was a stitch that looked like heavy black thread sticking out of my eyeball. I immediately felt dizzy, and everything started spinning. Lucky for me I live in a tiny house (purchased way before the whole tiny house movement) and was able to take two steps toward my bedroom and fall on the bed. I felt like Frankenstein, and I didn't know if the stitch was permanent or not. Would there always be a crude black thread sticking out of my eye? I cried. (And by the end of the next week, thankfully, the stitch had dissolved.)

I had regular checkups with the surgeon and usually one of my sisters would give me a ride. On one trip, as we drove down the street, I started to realize that my post-op vision was not so great. I saw a man carrying a baby in a car seat walking toward his car parked along the side of the street. I turned to my sister, "I can't believe that guy is carrying his baby that close to the road. He should put the car seat in from the other side!" "I totally agree," she said, "but that isn't a baby in a car seat, it's a toolbox." "Oh."

People from work called and stopped by with cards and gifts to lift my spirits. I told everyone I was doing as well as could be expected. I had issues with double vision since the scleral buckle was pushing the operated eye from its usual alignment, but there was a good chance that would resolve with time.

Christmas was approaching and luckily I had already done most of my Christmas shopping. My girls were able to spend extra time at their dad's house, which was helpful because I was unable to drive for the duration of my thirty-day recovery period. My man was able to come to town and that was nice. He didn't seem put off by my scary appearance and told me that he would always love me even if I lost the vision in both eyes. Good answer.

As December moved into January, I was anxious to reclaim my life and get back to work. I've always been a bit of a New Year's fanatic in that I truly believe that anything can happen in the new year and that it is most likely the beginning of the best year ever of my life. I also feel this way on every birthday. This year, the new year would be especially meaningful as the eye surgery would be behind me. I was now able to be up and about as much as I wanted as long as I didn't lift anything heavier than ten pounds, which is roughly the equivalent of a gallon of milk, or strain myself. Yes, the straining when constipated comment from my optometrist still haunted me.

On New Year's Day, I awoke and as I lay in bed and looked around, I suddenly thought that I saw "something" in the very top of my right eye, the operated eye. I called the surgeon's office right away. The answering service said they would relay my worries to the surgeon. He called and said he would see me the next morning. One of my sisters gave me a ride. (If you are getting the idea that I have a lot of sisters, you are correct. Four of them to be exact and one brother. His job is more 9 to 5, so while he offered moral support throughout the eye ordeal, it was usually a sister or my mom who provided transportation.) I was relieved when the surgeon said all was good and the retina was holding steady.

The recovery time dragged on, but soon, I was given the go ahead to return to work. I still patched the eye part of the time because the double vision had not resolved. So now I was out in the real world again and oftentimes wearing a patch. This is when I discovered that compared to other issues and health concerns, loss of vision and the wearing of a patch created a situation whereby levelheaded adults and others who you think would know better could not help themselves. Simply put, an eye patch equals humor. Sure, I expected this from snotty teenagers in stores who would notice the patch and poke their friends to make sure they also noticed. My balance was a bit off due to the lingering double vision, so sometimes I would misstep, or

13

wobble a bit, or try to return something to a store shelf and miss a bit or slam something down not realizing where the shelf was in relation to me. The teens would try to stifle a laugh and sometimes I would hear pirate noises made in my direction. I wanted to shake my finger at them and yell, "Hey, smart ass kids, go ahead and laugh, you'll be old someday too!" But I know teens don't really believe old age will ever happen to them, so I just ignored them.

The real surprise came from colleagues and other adults who you really think would know better. They don't know better. If you wear a patch, people cannot help themselves. "Hey, how much did the pirate pay for corn?" In case you don't know, the answer is a buck an ear. Get it? People would also ask me if it was Talk Like a Pirate Day. It was endless.

My first week back to work seemed okay. My boss was worried that it would be too much and asked me to limit myself to half time. This was fine, as the daily grind was exhausting. My girls were back at my house more of the time, so I appreciated not quite so much time at work, as getting two kids back and forth to school, plus homework help, and extracurricular activities felt like a lot. I tried to keep our house routine as simple as possible and didn't protest when someone wanted to drop off a meal or give the girls rides to and from school or to after school events.

By the end of my second week back to work, I kept thinking that I was seeing something, a shadow or something, at the top of my vision in my right eye. I called my surgeon's office, and his assistant said he was out of town for the next few days. I went home, and after lunch, I stood in front of my bathroom mirror brushing my teeth. I don't know why I did what I did next, because I hadn't yet read or heard about this tip to check your vision, but instinctively, I put one hand over my good eye. Now I know this is a recommended test for people who think they may have a vision issue. If part of your vision is missing, your brain will actually fill in the image and you may be totally unaware of the issue. I covered my good eye and looked in the mirror. "Oh my gosh!" I couldn't see anything above my shoulders, it was a dark curtain. I called the surgeon's office again. The receptionist suggested that I go see my regular eye doctor since the surgeon was out of town. I drove there immediately and told them I would see any available doctor. I, again, paid the extra $10 for the eye imaging. When the eye doctor got the results, he told me that, honestly, he wasn't a retina specialist and didn't know for sure what to recommend or what the scan was showing. He called my surgeon and together they decided that the best course of action was for me to go home and return to the post-surgery instructions of positioning and very little activity. The surgeon would see me first thing on Monday morning.

I tried to remain calm, but the weekend was filled with endless anxiety. Of course I was concerned about losing my vision, but as a working mom with high deductible insurance, I thought that this couldn't happen again. No way could I come up with my deductible again less than 30 days after the first surgery, which took place in the previous calendar year. I had already made arrangements with the hospital, the surgeon, and the anesthesiologist to make monthly payments to all three. No way could I get hit with another high deductible so soon. I called my insurance company with the hopeful question that a fiscal year would mean 365 days after the first incident. No luck, the calendar year was the fiscal year. The new year meant a new deductible to meet. This is one tip that everyone should know, if you have high deductible insurance and you have any choice at all in the scheduling of a major medical event (which I didn't) don't have surgery toward the end of the year. You can seriously get screwed if things go sideways.

I saw the surgeon on Monday morning, and he confirmed the worst. The retina was detaching again. I was devastated. I signed the papers for the next surgery, but even as I was signing, I knew I was done with this surgeon. Was the redetachment his fault? Was I to blame somehow? It didn't matter. As soon as I got home, I called the specialist eye center and told them my diagnosis. I was given an appointment the very next day. Then I called my man and my family members and shared the bad news while also asking who could give me a ride to the appointment. My girls packed up some things and I gave them a ride to their dad's house. The night was long and anxiety

15

filled. I tossed and turned. As I lay in bed, I made three vows to myself that this thing (the eye issue) would not become my life.

1. I wouldn't let it stop me from being a really good mom to my daughters.

2. I wouldn't let it drag down or end my relationship with my man.

3. And I would not let it take me down financially.

These vows to myself made me feel better. It didn't matter that I didn't know how I would make these three things happen. I finally went to sleep. The next day I got up super early to call my original surgeon's office to say that I would not be at the hospital at 6 a.m. for the emergency surgery and instead I would be seeing a specialist. Sure, that surgeon, his anesthesiologist, and the hospital would still be a part of my life for the next year or so as I made my monthly payments, but otherwise, I felt that I was on the cusp of better times for me and what I now openly referred to as my bad eye.

Chapter Two:
Surgery Two-Meet the Specialist

My sister who did laser work at the eye center gave me a ride the next day. I realized that I was feeling optimistic about the situation. I should mention that this same sister used to own dating service franchises. (She is a true entrepreneur and loves taking the risk to be her own boss. I admire that about her but have always loved my own work dedicated to public relations in the nonprofit sector. I love knowing that what I do every day makes life better for people in my community. She makes lives better too, just in a different way, like if someone was lonely and had trouble meeting people or if someone had facial or body hair that they don't want to deal with. Both of those situations can be remedied, and the results can be life changing.) She asked how my man was taking the news about the relapse. I told her he was totally supportive and had told me that even if I lost all my vision, he would still love me. "Well in case he doesn't, don't worry, I know for a fact that there are men out there who are totally open to meeting and dating women with physical challenges, including blindness." I wasn't sure how to take this. I wondered if she had encountered men in the dating service who were so amazing that they truly would and could see beyond physical differences? Or was she telling me about men with some sort of rescuing fixation that left them wanting to really, really help their partners? Or were there men out there who felt bad about their physical appearance and dating a blind woman would be a relief and spare them from any judgement or shame based on their looks?

The eye institute was the polar opposite of my first surgeon's office. It was huge, modern, clean, and beautifully designed. I was feeling better already. When I finally got to see the surgeon, he examined my eye closely. He confirmed the retina was detaching. It was a Tuesday, and his surgery day was Thursday. I would be added to the schedule. I signed the consent forms and asked him how to know if I was having an eye emergency before the surgery took place. He looked at me squarely and told me that nothing in that eye would be an emergency again. The central vision was lost over the weekend while I followed the advice of the first surgeon and the eye doctor. Hours counted at that point and the opportunity for saving the central vision was gone. "Wow!" The man did not mince words, and I was shocked but relieved to have someone tell me exactly what the situation was. I also asked him what could have caused the detachment. With zero hesitation, he said, "Age and nearsightedness." Okay, so 47 is old and a minus 4.5 of nearsightedness is enough to make this happen without any surprise on his part.

On Thursday, another sister (this one owns a ballet studio) drove me to the eye center for the surgery. Again, I was told not to eat or drink anything after midnight. So no coffee, no anything that morning. As we waited in the surgery center wing of the complex, my sister spied a fancy coffee bar for those who were waiting. Well, more accurately, for those who were family members or caregivers waiting on the patient. The patients could only smell the coffee. I looked daggers (or dagger since I only had one working eye) as she made herself a mocha latte while I sat in hunger and caffeine denial.

Finally, I was called back and prepped for surgery. One of the nurses explained the procedure to me. I would be put under but just for the first few minutes so they could put a numbing shot in my eye and complete the prep work (she didn't say that the prep would entail cutting off my eyelashes, clamping the eyelids wide open, and poking three holes in the eyeball, but that is part of the procedure.) Then I would come to and be awake during the surgery and most likely be aware of what was going on. "Wait. What...the... hell? Is this a joke?" I explained to her that I am extremely squeamish, and this wouldn't work at all. She assured me that I would be fine and that I couldn't be out during the actual surgery because if I were I might jerk or move involuntarily. I wasn't happy about it, but I had to agree.

A few minutes later, my surgeon came in and pulled a Sharpie from his pocket. He scribbled on my head above my right eye and told me he was marking the affected eye so that there would be no confusion in the operating room. As it turned out, I remained in the pre-surgery room for a while as he handled unexpected complications in the surgeries before mine. My sister was allowed to come back and wait with me. "What did he write on my face?" I asked her. She turned her head sideways to try to read the writing. "I'm not sure, but I think it says, 'I love you,'" she said. We both busted up laughing.

Before I knew it, I was being wheeled into the operating room. The anesthesiologist put me under, asking me to count backwards until I was out. A few minutes later I woke up. I heard music and felt confused. I could tell that my arms and legs were immobilized and felt pressure on my neck and head. Apparently, my face and neck were covered in a hood and were taped to the table and my arms and legs were swaddled tightly under the blankets so that I couldn't move. I lay there for a few seconds wondering if this was all real or not. I heard *This Old Heart of Mine* playing and noticed it was the original Isley Brothers version and not the remake with Rod Stewart and Ron Isley. "Why am I noticing this?" I thought to myself. At first, I couldn't "see" anything. My good eye was taped off along with the rest of my face. Only the operated eye was left uncovered, and the eyelids were being held back by surgical clamps keeping the eye extremely wide open. All I could see was a very bright light, but slowly I was able to see the shadow of the micro tools inside my eye as my surgeon worked. The surgery was a tri pars plana vitrectomy. Three holes are made in the eyeball and little, tiny tools are inserted. The first step is to suction out all of the vitreous fluid. Maybe I dreamed it, but I saw the outline of the tiny suction device as the fluid was drained from the eye. "Oh my gosh," I said out loud. The surgeon greeted me and told me what he was doing during each phase of the procedure. I laid there quietly wishing I didn't see the Monopoly-sized tools inside my head. Once he finished, an assistant ripped the tape off my face and neck, and I was wheeled into recovery. "Can I get you anything?" asked the nurse in the recovery room. "Maybe some therapy," I told her. My sister came in and I told her about the experience. When I told her I was awake and could see the tools inside my eye, she was horrified. "Why didn't you shut your eye?" she asked. It was hard to explain that the tools were literally inside my eye and there was no way to unsee them.

The eye was filled with saline to replace the original vitreous fluid, and an air bubble was also added to help hold the retina in place as it healed. I was given eye drops and the drop regimen along with instructions and the special foam pillow thing again so that I could position for the next several days. Maybe because this was a specialty eye center, the drops were already in a nifty little travel bag that also included wraparound sunglasses to protect my eyes.

Please know if you are facing eye surgery, there is no escaping the eye drop ritual. If you experience eye surgery, you will become somewhat of an expert about the many drops that are required. I felt that the prednisone drops made me sick to my stomach and maybe even more anxious than I normally am. I could feel the drops going down the back of my throat and taste them in my mouth. Most doctors and Google searches will tell you the prednisone drops do not cause system-wide reactions, but I'm not sure I believe this. If they are in your system, it seems that they will cause a reaction throughout your body. This may have been rationalization on my part, because during the course of the surgeries I started putting on some weight and I noticed the hair on my head getting thinner. I also started finding unexpected hairs popping up on my chin and upper lip. I wanted to blame it on something, but most likely it was perimenopause, and it would have happened with or without the eye drops.

At one point in my eye saga, and over the course of several months, the intraocular pressure (iop) went from really low to eventually really high, so glaucoma drops were needed. In stark contrast to the pred forte, these beta blocker drops are recognized as causing system-wide reactions, like hair loss, low blood pressure, and even heart failure. By that point however, I knew more about how to use eye drops more effectively, meaning as soon as you put the drop in your eye, you press a finger very firmly against the inner corner of the eye. This can stop the drop from draining to your sinuses and throat.

Because the vitrectomy surgery was less invasive than the scleral buckle surgery, my face wasn't nearly as bruised or swollen the next day. I felt optimistic throughout the required weeklong recovery and soon returned to work. But unfortunately, my saga was far from over.

Chapter Three:
Surgery Three-Not Again!

About four weeks after surgery number two, I had the sickening realization that I was seeing something again in my operated eye. The air bubble was shrinking like it was supposed to and I could see that I had some vision in the eye. But once again, a little shadow started to appear as the air bubble was dissipating.

"Are you kidding me?" I made an appointment with the surgeon and when I saw him a few days later he confirmed that the retina was once again detaching. How could this be? The surgeon told me that some people develop scarring issues. In fact, the scarring issue can be so pervasive that it is considered a disease in and of itself. It's called proliferative scarring. So surgery number three was scheduled. By this point, I was considered a frequent flyer at the surgery center. I preferred the term repeat offender because my recidivist eye refused to cooperate and behave as it should.

My eye doctor sister was incredulous, "Seriously, retina surgery is a one and done," she said. Apparently not for everyone. I started doing lots of internet searches and found lots of helpful information online. One favorite site was that of a retina surgeon on the east coast known as "The Retina Specialist." He maintains a very helpful website and blog and spends a lot of time responding to specific questions from people dealing with retina issues. One of his replies stuck with me regarding proliferative scarring. "Sometimes the disease wins," he said. Sad to read, but good to know the reality of the situation. I also learned that if one in ten thousand people get a detached retina, then two percent of those people develop proliferative scarring.

I also found myself spending time on a website called *Lost Eye*, which provides a forum for people who are losing vision in one or both eyes for a number of reasons. At first, I found the internet searches and the information helpful, but after a while, I felt like maybe all of the information was making me more anxious knowing all that could go wrong.

I asked my surgeon if the proliferative scarring was a sign of super healing, a term I learned during one of my internet searches. It's what happens more often with younger people. "No," he said. "You aren't that young." I laughed out loud because his matter-of-fact approach could be off-putting but was also exactly what I needed to hear.

When people found out I needed a third surgery, some would literally say to me, "It sucks to be you." I never agreed with this, but I didn't argue with anyone. The truth was, I was still a good mom with two amazing daughters, I was in a great relationship, and I had a job that I loved. And I still had my three vows to myself and hadn't failed myself yet and I was learning through necessity how to live as a single eyed person.

Surgery number three was mostly uneventful, except that to combat the tenacious scar tissue, the eye would be filled with saline, and a heavy gas bubble would be injected to keep the retina in place as it healed. At least this meant I did not have to position as much following the surgery because the gas bubble would do the work for me.

My man was able to be in town to take me to and from the surgery so that was especially nice to have him with me throughout the ordeal. I was fully in the second year of surgeries and with every surgery, I felt I was finally at the end of my vision saga.

But again, it was not meant to be.

Chapter Four:
Surgery Four-Cut it Out!

About four weeks after surgery number three, I felt certain that I was seeing something again in the vision. The gas bubble was getting smaller, like it was supposed to, but I was seeing something shadowy at the top of my vision again. My surgeon was sympathetic when he confirmed that indeed, the retina was trying to pull off again. He told me the next surgery would be more drastic. The part of my retina that kept detaching would be cut out (a retinotomy) and once the eye was emptied of the saline, it would instead be filled with heavy silicone oil. The silicone oil is a sign that all else has failed and a good visual outcome is probably not going to happen.

I was really unhappy to find out that I would need yet another surgery. "I would hate your job. Don't you ever give people good news?" I asked my surgeon. He didn't even look up as he said, "Sometimes we save lives and that is very rewarding."

"Crap." I forgot that the man is also an eye cancer specialist. He probably does save a lot of lives, especially young children with retinoblastoma, and yet he still has to listen to a bitchy almost 50-year-old who still has one good eye complain about another surgery.

And I know more about retinoblastoma, eye cancer, than I should. My ex-husband had Ewing's Sarcoma that started in his late teens (as it does for most people diagnosed with it) and he spent a considerable amount of time at Memorial Sloan Kettering Cancer Center in NYC. We had been dating for about a year when his cancer returned, and he went back to NYC for treatment. As soon as my spring semester was over, I bought a plane ticket and flew there to spend time with him. I had never flown before, and I had never been to NYC, but was surprised that it was fairly easy to navigate LaGuardia and to flag down taxis to get to and from the Ronald McDonald House in Manhattan where I stayed for my visit.

So many of the children there had retinoblastoma, or maybe it seemed like it because it is a cancer that you "see" immediately because of the eye patch. I never prayed so hard in my life, not only for my boyfriend's health but for every child I met and every parent whose

27

heart was breaking because their child was sick. I told my then-boyfriend that I never wanted to have children because if they ever got sick, really sick, I wouldn't be able to handle it. We actually waited several years after we married before we had kids. We wanted to feel confident that he would be around to help raise them and I had to come to terms with the risk that everyone takes when they become parents. It is exhausting and rewarding and a love like none you have ever known, but it can also break your heart.

So surgery number four was scheduled and took place just like the ones before it. The surgeon said the oil would really hold the retina in place and give it a chance to heal, and then usually six months later the oil is removed, and the eye is filled with saline and that could possibly improve the visual outcome.

One aspect of this particular surgery that struck me was the anesthesia or maybe it was the anesthesiologist. I was feeling like an old pro at the surgery procedure because, sadly, it had become a part of my life. In every surgery, the anesthesia was an unremarkable part of the procedure. But something was different in this surgery. The anesthesiologist was a female doctor. I didn't know if she had been a part of any of the previous surgeries, but what she did was magical. I went under like always, probably counting backwards until I was out and suddenly, I was totally and completely aware that I was experiencing the best, most wonderful, most restorative sleep of my entire life. I couldn't believe how wonderful it was and how lucky I was to be experiencing it.

Within a few minutes, I was awake again, listening to whatever music was playing and hearing any comments of the surgeon and the assistants. The surgery wrapped up, and as usual, the tape holding my head in place and the mask covering my face were ripped off. As I was being wheeled to the recovery room, I sat up and said, "Wait! I have to tell the anesthesiologist that I just had the most amazing sleep of my life! Thank you!" Everyone started laughing but I was totally serious.

Even now, years later, I think back to that feeling of rest and contentment that totally swallowed me for what was just a few minutes but somehow felt like it lasted a lifetime. It makes me wonder if I would be susceptible to drug use or abuse, because I think if I could find a way to feel what I felt that day, I would do it. Legally, of course.

Good reader, I wish I could tell you that surgery number four was the end of it, but sadly it was not. If you skip ahead, you will see that the surgery chapters continue. To warn you that there will be more, I will share a short story of when my ex-husband and I were newly married and went on double dates with other couples. We went to see *Four Weddings and a Funeral*. The title was odd to us and it was only after the first several minutes of the movie, when one wedding had taken place, that our friend whispered, "Crap, I get the title now, I guess we have to sit through three more of those and a funeral. Great!" I liked the movie, so I was not put off by his sudden realization. To be fair, anything with Hugh Grant usually gets my stamp of approval.

Anyway, this is all to say that after surgery number four, I was only halfway through the saga of saving what had become my mostly sightless eye. Given that, I could have titled this narrative *Eight Surgeries and a Bad Eye*, if I had wanted to give you a guide to what will follow. When I look back on the experiences now, I wonder for about a split second that if I knew that the eye would be sightless, would I still want to save it? But the question is ridiculous to me because every surgery was needed if I wanted to keep my eye. And I did want to keep it. Very much so, whether it was working or not.

Chapter Five:
Surgery Five-Hello Cataract

I should probably back up a bit to tell you that during my initial consultation with the eye center surgeon, he told me to expect a cataract to appear at some point due to the surgeries. "It might show up in two weeks or two years, but you will get a cataract as a result of the surgeries." And of course, with my bad eye, the cataract showed up sooner rather than later, within weeks of the fourth surgery, and would need to be removed, but not immediately.

As we approached the six-month mark of the oil being in place, my surgeon said the next surgery would need to take place to remove the cataract and to switch the oil to saline. (Yes, I heard a lot of oil change comments and jokes from my clever and funny coworkers.)

Apparently, if a cataract is not removed, it will grow and act like a sponge depriving the eye of needed fluids and it will destroy the eye. Sure, the eye was mostly non-functional as it was, but it was still my eye and I wanted to keep it. So surgery number five would be a two-part operation. The cataract surgeon was in the same eye center, so it would be seamless. The first part of the surgery would be the cataract removal and the second half would be my usual surgeon performing another tri pars plana vitrectomy to remove the oil and refill the eye with saline solution.

I know I have given you the impression that my regular surgeon is a no-nonsense kind of guy. Maybe I should also convey that he is highly regarded, highly sought out, and recognized for his research and his surgical skills. He is friendly, but also a man of few words. Whenever I was in the pre-surgery room, being tucked in with flannel sheets that were warmed in a dryer, I could tell the instant my surgeon was actually entering this part of the surgical wing. The usual chatter that I could halfway overhear as I waited would stop and I could hear a pin drop. That's when I knew he was in the hall and my surgery would be taking place soon. I told someone that it was like the Bugs Bunny cartoon where Bugs is Leopold, the adored yet feared, genius musical conductor. I never actually heard anyone whisper, "It's Leopold," but the hush that fell over the area was palpable.

31

When the two-part surgery took place, I was out for the first part while the cataract was removed. The last thing I remember was the cataract surgeon chatting with me before I was put under. He told me I had great teeth. I told him that while I was blessed with great teeth, apparently the tradeoff was a bad eye. I think we both laughed, but maybe it was operating room humor, where it really wouldn't have been funny anywhere else.

When the second part of the surgery started, I was out for a few minutes, as per usual, and then woke up. I was cognizant of the surgery and the activity in the room. "What is this?" I heard my retina surgeon say with disgust and impatience. A nervous voice said, "I thought I reset it to your specifications." "Not even close!" said my surgeon and an uncomfortable silence fell over the room. No usual music, no banter, just an uncomfortable silence. If I had been given a choice and if my head and neck had not been taped to the table and my arms and legs were not swaddled in such a way as to immobilize me, I would have climbed down from the table and crawled out of the room. But that wasn't an option, so the surgery continued, and the oil was siphoned out and the eye was refilled with saline solution.

Chapter Six:
Surgery Six-A Christmas Story

With surgery five behind me and the eye filled with saline, I looked forward to the possibility of some visual improvement. Surgery number five took place in early December and again, I felt like the coming new year could mean great things. Alas, the watery saline solution was no match for my retina and its propensity to detach again, even when it had been held down by the oil for the previous six months. Within two weeks and just a few days after Christmas, I was heading in for surgery number six. But this diagnosis had a slight wrinkle--and that is a really weak retina pun, because as the retina detaches over and over, it can be compared to a piece of aluminum foil (only much thinner and more delicate). As it falls and falls again, it becomes wrinkled and can never be smoothed out again with all of the rods and cones working together.

But this time the wrinkles weren't forming because of scarring issues. An ultrasound revealed that an epiretinal membrane was growing under the retina and it was pushing the retina up and causing it to detach again. My surgeon apologized to me and said he was sorry he did not realize sooner that a membrane had formed. Even as he was speaking, I remembered that I read somewhere that the number one reason why patients don't sue a doctor for malpractice is because the doctor says, "I'm sorry" when a situation could have possibly been avoided. I totally get that. I couldn't blame him for thinking the problem this time was the same problem it had always been, the proliferative scarring. The membrane would be removed, and the eye would be filled with oil. This surgery was also different in that I would be put under for the entire surgery. The surgeon knew it would be a difficult and deeper surgery than the others as he removed this epiretinal membrane. I thought this was great, because being awake during the surgeries was nerve-wracking. (But it wasn't great, the full anesthesia made me sick as a dog during the recovery process and I spent the next day and a half vomiting.)

On the day of the surgery, I went through the usual drill of being prepped for the surgery and then waiting in the pre-surgery room. This time, the waiting dragged on and on and my surgery was delayed considerably. As with any of my surgeries or even my checkups, I knew this was always a possibility. If things were running hours later than scheduled, I suspected that my surgeon was in surgery, probably saving the vision of someone in an emergency situation and whose vision still had the chance to be saved. Even though all of my surgeries were required to save the eyeball, the sight was pretty much long gone and as my surgeon told me early on, there wouldn't be any more emergencies for my bad eye.

At a post-op checkup a few days later, my surgeon told me the reason for the delay was that a little boy had been shot in the eye with a BB gun that he had gotten for Christmas. Unfortunately, the damage was too severe, and the little boy would lose his eye. I know right now you are thinking about *A Christmas Story*, and it is a funny movie, but sadly the cliché that everyone tells Ralphie that he can't have a BB gun because, "you'll put your eye out!" isn't an empty warning. Like lots of clichés, it is more of a truism, and it does happen.

Chapter Seven:
Surgery Seven-Wait, There's Another Word for Third?

At a post-op check about a month after surgery number six, my surgeon told me that my bad eye had wasted no time in developing a secondary cataract. Even though I could mostly just see lights and shadows in the eye, this secondary cataract would need to be removed, because just like the first one, it would destroy the eye. He would monitor its growth and schedule the surgery when it became too severe. He diagnosed the secondary cataract in January and surgery number seven was not required until August of that year.

It was a welcome respite. I was exhausted physically, emotionally, and financially from the endless surgeries. I was tired of knowing exactly how many Family Medical Leave Act days I had left in any given year. I was tired of saying no to trips and events that meant using time off from work that would be too precious in case yet another surgery was needed.

I wasn't excited about the prospect of one more surgery, but I knew it was required if I wanted to keep my eye. And even though it was mostly worthless, it was still my eye and I wanted it in my head. When I told my coworkers about it, I tried to be positive. "Apparently I have a secondary cataract," I said. "I know that has to be the end of this eye saga because it's a secondary cataract and I don't think there's a word for a third time of something," I joked in a meeting. Immediately, at least a half a dozen people shouted out the word, "tertiary" like they were on *Jeopardy* or in a trivia contest at a bar. "Of course," I thought, "that's what happens when you work with really smart people." I took a ton of Latin and Greek classes in high school and college, but I swear I did not learn or remember the word tertiary. At one point, I found myself accidentally enrolled in a Bio Scientific Latin and Greek terminology class. Apparently, it was intended for those going into medical fields. The highlight of the class, for me, was learning there was a medical term for throwing up poop, copremesis. Maybe if tertiary described something so horrifying as throwing up poop, I would have remembered it. So, surgery number seven took place and the secondary cataract was removed and the eye was refilled with oil. My surgeon said even though oil is generally removed after six months, for some people, like me, it would just stay there indefinitely. I was okay with this. I Googled about what happens if the silicone oil stays in the eye forever and found one unfortunate story about the oil migrating out of the eye and into the patient's brain or head, or something equally alarming. I immediately stopped reading and decided to never do that Google search again.

As I mentioned earlier, the standard visitor to the surgery center is an older person often being helped by a younger person. At one of my checkups following this surgery, I was accompanied, as I often was, by my mom. We were leaving a post-surgery checkup. My bad eye was patched, and wonder of wonders, at the end of a long hallway walking toward us was a younger man, probably about my age, wearing a patch, and he was accompanied by an older man, probably his father.

I know I might be prone to flights of fancy, and yes, I am in a great relationship, but I swear that his single eye locked vision with my single eye. We both got it and acknowledged the situation with a slight nod. His left eye was patched, and my right eye was patched. Individually, we were sight-impaired, but together maybe we could rule the peripheral world! I thought about it later, was this a James Blunt moment? Were we destined to be together, but just walked on by? Probably not, but sometimes you just have to wonder why the universe puts us where we are at a certain time and place.

It made me think about the time I read *Candy Freak* by Steve Almond. I am a candy freak and couldn't believe that this writer experienced candy and appreciated it on a level that only other candy freaks can appreciate. "Who is this man and why didn't the universe conspire to bring us together?" I thought while reading the book and eating candy. I flipped the book over to stare at Almond's picture and read his bio. "Hmmmm." Although Almond was younger, he bore a striking resemblance to my ex-husband and he also taught writing at a university, just like my ex-husband. "Hmmmm, maybe the universe did conspire to put a man very much like him in my orbit and it didn't work out," I thought.

Maybe the universe knows what it is doing. Maybe the outcome would have been disappointing with the younger man patient I saw at the surgery center. Maybe being roughly the same age and dealing with a similar vision issue would not guarantee compatibility. Maybe James Blunt's angel on the subway was physically beautiful but actually really annoying in daily life. Maybe Blunt should have considered this possibility before diving to his music video death.

Chapter Eight:
Surgery Eight-A Hole in the Story

If there are maxims in the eye care world like, "one and done" for retina surgeries, then another given is that a retina will not detach in the presence of heavy silicone oil. So it was very upsetting when about four weeks after the surgery and the silicone oil fill that I was quite certain I was seeing something again in the bad eye. I called my eye doctor sister and she assured me, "That never happens, well, very rarely," she said.

I got off the phone and stayed up all night watching the activity in my bad eye. I could see line after line falling into place and forming a weird network of shapes and lines in the eye.

This is really hard to explain to anyone, but the bad eye filled with oil could really only see lights. If I was in a darkened room and covered my good eye, I would know if a light was on because I would see a faint glow and if something was in front of the light like a hand, I could see its silhouette. But here is where it gets really weird, because there are other things the bad eye can see, things that aren't really there, but that I see across my entire span of vision. Like moving silhouettes of shapes and such across my brain. It's like a cloud with splotches of darkness and patches of less darkness swirling and moving about. I had grown as used to this as one possibly can. And since I need to work in gainful employment, I just try to ignore it.

Okay, I Googled this visual phenomena and found that it usually only happens to people who have sustained serious eye damage and to people using LSD. People also see grids, patterns, and other visual phenomena. This is totally different from floaters and this onslaught of visual snow can cause anxiety and depression in some. "Great."

Anyway, a visit to the surgery center revealed that the retina, while holding in place, now had a hole in it. The hole was adding to the weird visual phenomena. Surgery would be needed to repair the hole and then, of course, the eye would be refilled with heavy oil.

41

I have to come clean that at some point, even though I remained compliant about the surgeries, I became a bit more relaxed about the pre-surgery instructions. By this, I mean I stashed Reese's peanut butter cups in my purse and would visit the restroom right before I was called back to the surgery wing, so I could eat a few. I've always been a three-square meals kind of girl and the whole "not eating after midnight" thing was too hard. I decided if I were to choke and aspirate during the surgery, it would be on my terms and it would involve chocolate.

This cavalier attitude did not serve me well for surgery number eight. This time, I went so far as to have a cup of coffee at my house before my mom came to drive me to the surgery center. I knew it was wrong, but I felt like I really needed it. Unfortunately, the surgery took longer than the usual surgery. Yes, I went to the bathroom and peed before I was wheeled into the operating room, but the surgery dragged on and after a while I really had to pee.

"How are you doing?" asked the surgeon. "I need to pee," I told him. "Well, that isn't possible," he replied as he continued his work. A while later he asked, "Are you doing okay?" "I still need to pee," I said. What I didn't say out loud, but that I wanted to rant was, "Come on, we can put a man on the moon, but I can't have a catheter or a bedpan!" So, I had to lay there in agony. And as an almost fifty-year-old woman with plenty of pelvic prolapse issues from having Large Marge babies, it really was agony.

I wondered why they couldn't cath me. Surely, this wasn't the first time it ever came up in one of these surgeries. I thought about a coworker friend, one of our children's librarians, who had shown me a printable coloring page one of our young customers had colored for her. It was the Gingerbread Man in full sprint mode with a typo in the caption. "Cath me if you can!" "What the hell Mr. Gingerbread Man?" she said as she showed me the artwork. "Do you even have a urethra?" Thinking about this made me feel a little better and I survived the surgery and peed like a racehorse as soon as I got to the recovery room bathroom. So, lesson learned about coffee prior to surgery! Although it was my final surgery, so fingers crossed that I never have the opportunity to use that hard-learned lesson.

Chapter Nine:
Random Thoughts and Questions That May or May Not Help Others

If you have read this far, I thank you and suspect that maybe you have experienced visual loss or have had eye surgery or several eye surgeries. Like me, you may have found that there is some information on the internet but not a lot of support to help us to understand or navigate our newly sight-impaired world. One oddity I have noticed in internet searches of my eye diagnoses or prescribed medications is that the first or second results of the search pertain to humans and then it quickly devolves to veterinary medicine involving cataracts in dogs and eye drop tolerance in dogs. I'm not sure how to take this.

In this chapter, I will attempt to share observations, offer some suggestions that have helped me maintain some semblance of a normal life, and answer some important questions that may arise.

Will I develop a crush on my surgeon? (asking for a friend) Okay, with apologies to my man, I have to confess that this is a thing. And I can only speak from my own experience, but I feel this is fairly common. If you think about it, your surgeon becomes one of the most important people in your life. You are scared and have questions, he or she has the answers. In the most stressful situations in the operating room, his or her voice is commanding and calm. I don't know if crush is the right way to describe it, but definitely the halo effect will be in full force.

When I found out the wife of a university professor I was collaborating with for a library program was also a patient of my surgeon, I gushed about how fortunate I was to be under his care. "He is THE MAN!" the professor nearly shouted, which made me think that maybe even some guy crushes develop and unless this admiration is taken to the extreme, most patients and their significant others will not become stalkers but will generally hold the surgeon in a place of high esteem. It is natural.

How to not become pain pill addicted. I didn't really think much about this until I watched a PBS documentary that featured stories of people who were pretty much minding their own business and living their lives when an accident or other medical event took place. Within a year or so of major surgery, the individuals became addicted to pain medications and opioids and their lives spun out of control. Lost jobs, broken families, bankruptcy, illegal activities, incarceration, and accidental or intentional fatal overdoses followed. I thought about this in the context of my own surgeries over the course of three years and I became very grateful for the surgeons I had. Both were extremely stingy with any pain medication and while I might not have appreciated this fully at first, I could see the reasoning that was at work. Many of their patients were probably a bit older than me—maybe in their fifties, sixties, seventies, and beyond. I'm sure any age group could be susceptible to overuse of pain medication, but maybe an older population could be even more vulnerable. I remember being at a party and someone jokingly asked if I had a stash of serious pain meds from all of the surgeries. I said no, and that the only pain medication prescribed was Tylenol 3, and even then, it was only enough for one or two days following the surgery. A doctor at the party said, "Wow, your surgeon must hate you!" Everyone laughed, but later I thought that actually the surgeons I worked with maybe had already seen enough lives ruined by pain pill addiction. They weren't going to let any patients get sucked into that downward spiral on their watch. So if you are given prescriptions for pain medications, use them sparingly or even ask for the lowest strength possible or even consider over-the-counter pain meds.

Visual disturbances. Floaters can happen at any time but generally they happen when one's vitreous gel in the eye liquefies and pulls away from the retina. This happens naturally as part of the aging process, maybe in one's fifties. Usually this happens with no major incident, but in some cases, as with mine, part of the retina stuck to the gel as it liquefied, and this is probably what caused the initial detachment. The other thing that can happen is that floaters are formed. These are strands of protein that swirl around in the liquefied vitreous and are seen as squiggles and blobs that block your vision. So, while my good eye has good vision, it also has several floaters that I notice especially when looking at a blank wall, a ceiling, or when looking at the sky. They are super annoying but thankfully don't generally indicate that something more serious is happening. Once you have them, they don't go away, you just get more used to them.

I have an odd assortment of specks and blobs in my good eye that I have learned to live with. I call one of them Kibbles and Bits because it is a two-part floater with a bigger and more blobbish bit that moves slowly, and a smaller, more intense spot that seems tied to the bigger blob. The small dot kind of jumps around the larger blob as it lumbers through my vision whenever I move my eye. It reminds me of the dog food commercial with the big English bulldog marching across the screen with a much smaller, skittish Jack Russell hopping up and down at his side.

Another frustrating outcome that can't be measured on an eye chart, are the visual disturbances and anomalies that many eye surgery patients experience. This became more of a thing for me following the oil-filled surgeries. My own theory is that the oil acts on or creates physical pressure on the poor confused rods and cones and this creates a lot of crap in my vision from inside my eye and inside my brain. For this reason, it doesn't matter if one or two eyes are opened or closed. It is a nearly constant visual barrage that is happening inside my head and as far as I know, there isn't anything that can be done to fix it.

This is the visual phenomena I mentioned earlier, which increased when the retina had a hole in it, but which has lessened in intensity once the hole was repaired, but that has never gone away in the ten years that have passed since the last surgery. One form of it is called Charles Bonnet Syndrome and it happens mostly in older people with macular degeneration and diabetic retinopathy. Wikipedia says that "They experience hallucinations as the brain adjusts to significant vision loss. The hallucinations can be simple geometric patterns, or much more complex scenes involving animals, people and places." Mine are not elaborate, no animal or people hallucinations, just a steady swirl of geometric patterns, spinning fans, and patchy clouds pulsating across my brain. All day. Every day. It's called visual snow and there are some pretty good pictures online that represent what this looks like. To me. Inside my own head. All day. Every day.

Another visual anomaly that started after my first cataract was removed was a cannonball of light that would swoop in from the outside edge of my bad eye and swirl around a bit and then shoot out of my range of vision. These lights are random but seem to happen more if I move my head suddenly or change position. Again, no one else can see this. It's just inside my head.

If you are getting the idea that it takes some amount of fortitude to remain sane, act normal, and continue to be employed as a sight-impaired person with one eye and constant visual disturbances, you are correct. There is very little support, and I don't even know if there is a profession dedicated to helping us. How can someone help you deal with visual crap no one else can see? My surgeon's chief concern when I see him is the condition of the retina. Is it holding in the bad eye? And is the retina in the good eye still good? This is his specialty, and he is an expert at it. I admire him greatly. But he can't offer much assistance in dealing with how to navigate visual impairment.

During one of the surgeries mentioned earlier, the oil was removed after six months, and the bad eye was refilled with saline solution. But all of the oil can't be removed, no matter how skilled the surgeon. A bit of oil will remain and when the eye is filled with saline, the patient will have and will see a bubble of oil floating in that eye. Forever. It's like having a carpenter's level or a lava lamp in front of you at all times. I guess it is worth the trade off if the saline gives the patient a better visual outcome. I remember asking my surgeon about it at a post-op appointment. "How do people deal with this bubble in their vision?" In true form, my surgeon replied, "They deal with it." To be honest, it was almost a relief when the retina detached again and the eye was refilled with oil (and would remain oil filled) and the bubble went away.

Dear reader, if you have that bubble in your vision or experience the visual disturbances and visual snow that I have described, you have my sympathy, and I can only suggest that you do your best to ignore it. With time, you will be able to continue speaking and working even when a cannon ball of light is passing through your vision. Know that it will make you a bit more distracted than you used to be. When I was younger, one of my frequent New Year's resolutions was to not finish sentences for other people. It's rude. Yes, I am a word nerd, and I probably do know the word you might be searching for, but I should not finish your sentences for you.

Ironically, because of the visual distractions or maybe just because I am getting older, I now have trouble sometimes finishing my own damn sentences. Is it the result of the visual phenomena, or is it just karma payback for years of finishing sentences for others?

How do I navigate my workplace? In the U.S. at least, single eye vision is recognized as a sight-impairment, but in most cases, the person's vision and prospects for employability are as good as the vision in the good eye. So if your good eye, with glasses or contacts, provides decent enough vision, you are good to go. Of course, for many of us, the good eye may see the letters on the chart just fine, but the eye test doesn't take into account the floaters and other visual disturbances that may be bouncing around in the vision.

Assuming that you need to work, and most of us do, here are a few suggestions for your workplace. Rearrange your office so that people approach from your good side. Sit at meetings so that people are on your good side. At seminars and conferences, sit at whichever far side of the room allows you to see most of the room. Try to control where you are sitting so that most of the action takes place on your good side.

Can I drive? Good question. And only you can decide what the answer is. I don't drive on the highway anymore. My surgeon didn't tell me I couldn't drive on the highway, but I decided that too much happens on the right side, like merging, exit signs, ramps, etc. for me to be comfortable with it. Obviously, if your left eye is bad or if you live in the United Kingdom, these details may be reversed. Even driving around town and to and from work can be challenging and I make every attempt to be overly vigilant and to not cause harm to myself or others.

As it turned out, my driver's license expired at about the same time as my last surgery. I was a bit nervous about having it renewed. An eye test would most likely be a part of the renewal process. I decided that if I were denied a license, it would be a real hardship, but I would have to agree with whatever the Bureau of Motor Vehicles felt was in the best interest of public safety. Still, I decided when I took the eye test I would do my best to use my good eye to cover for the visual loss in my bad eye. I know, I'm not proud to admit this, but I had every intention of cheating.

When it came time for the test, the good eye passed just fine. The BMV rep then switched something on the machine to test my right eye and said, "Read the smallest line you can read." I couldn't see any lines. It was all dark. Nothing. Apparently, there is an impenetrable separation within the machine so that a person can't cheat and look over with a good eye to try to see anything. "Rats!" After an uncomfortable silence, I told the BMV rep that I couldn't see anything and was there a chance the machine was broken? She marched out from behind the counter and peered into the machine. "This unit is working just fine," she said. "Oh." I came clean and told her that my right eye was basically blind. She reassured me that at least in Indiana, this was not an issue and I could still be granted a driver's license. The only drawback was that I could not be licensed as a commercial driver. Not a big deal to me, but for someone who needs a CDL, this could be horrible news.

Following the surgeries, several people told me they had family members who had single eye vision who had decided to never drive again at all. I understand that. It can be hard.

I always make sure there are no leaves or anything on my windshield. My brain knows it is a leaf, but sometimes it's as if a zoom lens takes over when you don't have three-dimensional vision, and the leaf might still be a little leaf about two feet away from you stuck to the windshield but suddenly it looks like a dog or a person standing along the curb. It's freaky. Size and space perception can be off. Way off.

Even two-way stops can be hazardous. It takes more time than you think to see that the road is clear to your left and then turn your head entirely to the right to see that nothing is coming from that direction either. A lot can happen in that extra second or two. When I first started driving again, I found myself saying, "I didn't see that coming," more than once. One defensive move I have taken is that I mostly drive on roads that I know, and I try to use roads that have four-way stops and stop lights. So, if everyone follows the rules, I get my turn and don't have to feel at risk of a car surprising me because of those extra seconds it takes to look both ways.

Another good tip for driving is to find and shop at stores that have parking spaces where you can pull through the space. Why doesn't everyone do this? It's genius. Now, you never have to back out of a parking space. And while I'm at it, if possible and if you are experiencing any dizziness as you acclimate to your single eye vision, park close to a cart corral. You are pushing a cart, just like everybody else, and if you are a bit disoriented, the cart steadies you, so it's nobody's business but your own.

Drive up windows, ATMs, and mail drop boxes can also be very difficult. It is so hard to see how close you are. Just take it slow.

Living 2-D in a 3-D world. It was surprising to me and it surprises others to learn that if you don't have two eyes, you don't really have 3-D vision anymore. It takes visual input from both eyes for the brain to create the 3-D effect. So when walking and while driving, extra care and caution are needed.

You learn there are other visual cues that can help, like shadows, painted curbs, edge strips on steps, puddles, and things like that. These cues let you know that something is a step up or maybe that a sidewalk is on an incline.

I remember one Christmas after losing my vision, I got one of my daughters a Nintendo 3-D. I was so excited for her to open it because

I wanted to test my 3-Dness. It was pretty disappointing that it did not look 3-D to me at all. However, when she demonstrated the AR (augmented reality) cards that came with it, I did feel amazed to see Mario appear to hop off the card and run around on the table when I viewed it through the gaming device.

I also get a real sense of 3-D when I visit the planetarium at the local university. For some reason when I lean back in the totally dark room and see the star formations projected on the screen, I get a sense of depth perception. I know I don't have 3-D vision, but in the dark planetarium I kind of, sort of, feel like I do.

Lack of 3-D vision also means relearning a lot of everyday activities. What should you do when pouring coffee or other drinks at home or, God forbid, you are at a luncheon or other event, and someone asks you to pour something for them? Honestly, sometimes I will just say, "You don't want me to do that." But obviously you have to relearn to pour things to function. So do this. Keep the glass or coffee cup on the table. Hold onto the glass with one hand (that tells your brain where it is) and put the lip of the carafe or the pitcher right against the rim of the glass or cup. Of course, people who know me never ask me to pour things. They know it is stressful and doesn't always end well.

A friend and I meet sometimes at a fast-food restaurant for a quick lunch that is usually more talking than eating, but when the place added a new self-serve Coke machine with a touch screen, it was too much. After one or two episodes of me thinking the cup was on the target, but it wasn't quite aligned or me thinking I was pushing one button on the touch screen, but hitting a different virtual button, I gave up. I always ended up with my sleeves soaked in pop and the cup semi-filled with something other than what I thought I had poured. Thankfully, my friend graciously always offers to get my drinks for me.

Yet, oddly enough, the people closest to you may seem to forget that your visual world is different. For some reason, ever since my stepfather passed away a few years ago, I am always tapped to carve the ham or turkey, or whatever large hunk of meat my family is having at get togethers. "Really? You just got a new set of razor-sharp knives from QVC and you think it's a good idea for the sight-impaired girl to use them?" Even worse, my stepdad always used an electric carving knife that was returned to its original box after each use and the first time I was in charge of the meat carving, my mom was upset because she couldn't find it. "Really? You want the sight-impaired girl to use a pulsating power knife to carve the meat?"

Ladders also deserve a mention in regard to not having 3-D vision. In general, if you can avoid them, do so. But this isn't always possible. I have learned the hard way that the trick is to not look down as you climb down the ladder. You will think that you are closer to the ground than you are and you will take that final step expecting your foot to connect with solid ground and it won't. You will tumble. So don't look down, just keep climbing down rung by rung until you actually feel your foot touch the ground. Problem solved. Getting toothpaste onto the toothbrush and putting keys in locks can also take some practice but you will get better at it. The clear steps at the Apple store in Manhattan? Please avoid! I only felt safe navigating these because I was there on a Friday, the day after the July 4 holiday and everyone was apparently off work and in Manhattan. I felt that if I did fall, I would have landed on top of a bunch of other tourists and the injury would have been minimal.

Eye patches. Another thought I will share is about the use of an eye patch. Yes, many of us have to wear one after surgery and for people who lose their eye or are left with seriously disorienting vision, a patch can offer relief. People were surprised when I started wearing glasses again after all of my surgeries, instead of the contacts I had worn most of my adult life. "You should wear your contacts (well, one contact since there is no point of vision correction in the blind eye) and a patch on your bad eye. It would look so cool," people told me more than once. I agree, an eye patch can look quite roguish and dashing on men and women, but please take a minute to think about the situation.

The patch is covering the bad eye, which means the person has exactly one good eye left. And in many cases, the vision in the "good" eye isn't all that good. On top of this, single eye vision means no peripheral vision, depth perception, and little chance to see if one is about to get beaned by an errant ball or smacked by a branch from a tree or bush you might be trimming. There is just too much that can go wrong. One of my surgeon's assistants pointed this out to me and it made perfect sense. She said they really prefer that patients have the protection of glasses covering both eyes at all times. Even, or especially, when you get up to use the bathroom in the middle of the night. She said patients who had been left with vision in one eye had experienced tripping or falling accidents at home and now the vision was gone from the good eye too.

Glasses. Here's a thought about ordering glasses. If one eye is totally blind and it can't be corrected, order the lens for that side of your glasses in the exact same strength as the lens for the good eye. Why? Because the prescription, especially if it is strong, will change how others see your eye. If one lens is a minus 4.5 of nearsightedness and the other lens is clear, there will be a noticeable difference in the appearance of one eye when compared to the other. Okay, there will be some differences anyway, but at least give your face a fighting chance to look normal. Also, don't get the special anti-glare coatings. Let those lenses be perfectly shiny so people are less aware of the differences in the two eyes. I'm not suggesting that looking like one of the round-headed laboratory scientists from *The Muppet Show* should be your face goal, but shiny lenses can help camouflage the noticeable differences.

Droop along. Some patients will have ptosis following an eye surgery or multiple eye surgeries. Ptosis is when the eyelid droops and the muscles that used to hold the eye open no longer work quite as well. Think about it, the eyelid gets clipped back with surgical clamps during the surgery and this can be very damaging. I have to give kudos to the surgery teams I worked with that I have very little eyelid drooping, even after eight surgeries. Although I am loath to consider any further surgeries, if my eyelid develops a noticeable droop, I probably will consider surgery to repair it. For some reason eyelid surgery seems less horrific than eyeball surgery.

Becoming a walleye. Something else that you may not know that I didn't know until after losing all vision in my right eye, is that a blind eye won't look at things and track in unison with your good eye. I know, haven't we suffered enough? I was totally pissed off when this truth became known to me. I was at work discussing an upcoming event with one of our program planners. He paused mid-sentence and turned his head quickly to the left to see what I was looking at in the right corner of my office. I wasn't looking at anything in the right corner but apparently my bad eye was!

I asked my surgeon about this the next time I saw him. "Yes, this is part of the process. The eye can't see anything, so the brain rejects any input from that eye. So now the eye will wander," he said. I had never heard of this and was shocked. I didn't want to become a walleye (which is a horrible term, I know, and I'm pretty sure it comes from a walleye fish.) How can life be so damn cruel? Is it not enough that losing the vision changes how I see? Now it also gets to change how I look. Yes, I realize that this makes me sound petty. I should rejoice in the vision I still have, and I do, but sometimes this whole process can provoke some self-pity and I think that is only natural.

I told my eye doctor sister that I planned to overcome this issue with nightly eye exercises. The eye could still see light, so I would shut off the lights, squeeze my good eye shut, and make my bad eye follow a flashlight beam to see if that visual input would be enough to keep the eye aligned with the good one and enough input for the brain to value the bad eye's contributions. She wasn't impressed with my plan and broke the news that it wouldn't do any good. "Rats!" Instead, she suggested, as my surgeon had, that if the eye became too misaligned, I could undergo an outpatient procedure that I think involved some sort of surgical tether or cord that could pull the eye in the right direction. Seriously, this sounded too horrible to consider. My man agreed. "Fuck that. If your eye gets too bad and you feel self-conscious about it, you can start wearing dark glasses," he said. Again, good answer.

Ch,ch,changes. So ten years later the eye does drift sometimes. Not always. I haven't switched to dark glasses yet, but it is still a possibility as my eye developed another complication that I can't remember the name of. It has something to do with the pigment in my bad eye and the scarring that was created by the scleral buckle that remains stitched onto the back of my eye.

I was out of town at my man's house getting ready in the morning. The lighting was different from my usual get ready routine at my own house. A window in the room was flooding the right side of my face with sunlight and I did a double take as I looked at my bad eye. I couldn't believe that all along the edges of my blue iris was a wavy ring of gold that was almost yellow. "What is that and why am I just noticing it?" I was able to visit my surgeon a few days later when I got back to Indiana. I was so scared because I thought, "After all of this, I am still going to lose this eye." The thought of a glass eye makes me really squeamish. I don't say this to insult or hurt the feelings of anyone with a glass eye. I think they look fine and can be made to match the good eye and often can appear to track and move naturally with the good eye. It's just that I don't want one. I think it would be too much for my squeamish self to deal with.

Thankfully, my surgeon said it was nothing to be concerned about, so that was a huge relief. However, the gold circle continued to grow wider and cover more of my blue. It also seemed to move inwards just a bit month by month to the center of the eye. So now it is like a gold bullseye around the pupil and the pupil itself looks like there is a cloudy, gold hue to the formerly dark dot. I take super close-up selfies of it every few weeks just to monitor its change. My surgeon didn't ask me to do this, but for some reason, I want to know what it is doing. I joke with his assistants that if the ring of color continues to grow, I will end up either looking like a cyborg or possibly David Bowie with two different colored eyes (yeah, I know, wishful thinking, as if anybody else could look that cool.)

Word choices. I have to share that having vision issues and becoming sight-impaired and having an interest in words and writing which is to be expected because I have a journalism degree, I became almost hyper-aware of all of the terms and phrases that all of us use a million times a day that have to do with sight. People in my family always say "Ask Susan" if there is a question about paint chips or decorating. "She has an eye for it." (So does another sister, who has a fine arts degree and works as an art teacher and an interior designer. But she lives out of state, so I am the resident expert.) But yes, I do have an eye for it, exactly one eye for color choice and design ideas. People at work would ask me to keep an eye on a situation and then would get flustered realizing that I had exactly one eye to do the job. Hindsight is 20/20. Is it if you only have one eye? Is it easier for me to turn a blind eye now that I have one? Do you see what I mean? Exactly.

Another word observation I made as I went through surgery after surgery, always with the secret hope that my vision would be restored, but armed with the reality that it wouldn't be, was the way people described me. I was told by others over and over that I was brave. I know people said this as a way of being kind and supportive but I found this word choice odd and I never felt brave. I may have a different take on people (patients) being labeled as brave. In my own mind and in my situation, the word compliant was the more apt description. I was simply compliant every time a surgery was needed to save the eyeball. I complied when asked to sign the surgery consent forms, I complied when I showed up on the day of the surgery, and I complied when told to strip down and don a surgery gown, climb up on the operating table, and wait to be wheeled into the operating room. I didn't feel brave. I felt compliant. (Except, of course, when I ate chocolate or drank coffee prior to the surgeries.)

Woulda, shoulda, coulda. One woulda, shoulda, coulda that came up during my eye saga was that I had not requested dilated exams at my annual eye appointments. My boss at the time was incredulous that I didn't know to do this. She had a minus 10 nearsightedness, which is a really strong prescription, and she always had dilated exams so her retinas could be evaluated. My prescription was only a minus 4.5, which isn't nearly as hyper myopic. Yet in hindsight, I wish I had known to do this. My eye doctor sister told me not to sweat it, even though she generally conducted dilated exams on any of her patients with elevated nearsightedness. "It doesn't always help," she said. "I've done fully dilated exams and a patient's retinas looked fine and yet more than once, a spontaneous detachment happened within a month."

I think everyone thinks back over their life and wonders about other wouldas and shouldas, and if choices we made were right or wrong.

Even though my family moved around a lot as I was growing up, we always returned to Muncie, Indiana. I think it was because my mom's extended family lives here, so it made sense. I ended up graduating from a high school that is affiliated with Ball State University (named after the Ball Brothers who made Ball jars, in case you were wondering. David Letterman is one of BSU's most famous graduates. Muncie is also famous for Garfield the Cat, who I love and think is hilarious--and not ironically. His creator, Jim Davis, is amazingly generous and my library system is grateful for this.) The high school is in a beautiful older building on the campus. The original quad part of campus is filled with other beautiful old buildings, and the rest of campus is beautiful too. But the point is, I went to high school here and then to college here. And now I live about a mile from the center of campus. And I love the campus, but sometimes when I'm sitting at a stoplight on campus, I look to my right (which requires me to totally turn my head, since I can only see with my left eye) and I see my high school. I look to the left and see the BSU Administration Building and even though I think I am happy with the choices I have made in my life, I can't help but think that at least geographically speaking, I didn't get very far.

A thought related to this that crept into my mind after my eye surgery experiences is that my serious boyfriend in high school went on to become an eye doctor. It makes me think, what if we would have stayed together? What if I had been married to an eye doctor? Maybe when I told him about the little squiggly thing in my vision, he would have rushed me to a specialist and my eye story would have been the one and done surgery like it is for almost everyone else. It might have saved my vision.

I don't spend a lot of time thinking about this or other wouldas and couldas because the fact of the matter is that he dumped me, so it's not as if a choice I made lots of years ago would have made a difference now. Maybe whoever Mrs. Eye Doctor is will be the recipient of this hidden benefit of being married to him if she ever develops a spontaneous detached retina. (Or maybe she is an eye doctor too, who knows?) At any rate, good for her.

Privilege. I would be remiss if I did not address the fact that I am beyond privileged to have had access to good medical care throughout my eye saga. I am ashamed to say that I didn't even consider this privileged status while I was in the thick of losing my vision. This awareness came to me very suddenly when I met someone who did not have the same opportunities.

I was driving back to work after lunch one day. At this point, the bad eye was its usual bad self but I was, at least temporarily, in between surgeries. My car had a very unreliable gas gauge that gave the low gas warning randomly. I usually just reset the trip meter whenever I filled up and never had an issue. Well, the low gas warning was on and I noticed from the trip meter that I probably was actually really close to running out of gas. Did I stop immediately to fill up? No, I kept driving because I wanted to get to a gas station closest to my office that charges two cents less per gallon. I was shocked when my car died at an intersection about a block away from the gas station. Luckily, there was an auto repair shop right on the corner. I walked into the bay where a mechanic was working on a vehicle and asked if I could borrow one of the gas cans lined up along the wall. He said it was no problem and that he was sorry he couldn't give me a ride to the closest station but he was the only one there and no one else could watch the shop. Since we both could literally see the sign for the gas station I was trying to get to, I assured him that I was fine to walk the necessary block to get it myself.

I got the gas and started my car and pulled in to the repair shop's parking lot to return the gas can. The mechanic was standing outside the bay and as I handed the gas can to him while saying thanks, I misjudged how close we were. I offered the can in his general direction, and he fumbled to take it from me. I'm sure to anyone driving by it looked like we were playing hot potato with the can as it wobbled clumsily between us. I apologized and told him I was newly sight-impaired and was having a lot of trouble figuring out my distance in relation to pretty much everything. He laughed and told me he was sight-impaired too. It turns out he was injured in a bar fight, and he was losing the vision in one eye.

I ran back to my car to get my surgeon's business card to give him. I told him that if there was any chance to save any of the vision, my surgeon was the person to do it. I still remember the look he gave me as he shook his head. "I don't have insurance," he said. "Whatever is going to happen to my eye, is going to happen." I was immediately embarrassed and ashamed of my presumption that everyone with a health problem could reach out and get health care if they wanted it. Yes, coming up with the annual deductible for high deductible insurance for several years in a row was hard. But it must be much harder to lose your vision because you don't have the means to at least try to save it because you don't have insurance.

Later, I told my man about the encounter and wondered if I could find an organization or other resource to let the mechanic know about. "Let it go," he said to me. "You can't fix everyone's life and probably you will just give him false hope." I knew he was right. But it makes me sad that sometimes the disease wins and that sometimes other crappy outcomes get to win too. Why should I have the opportunity to try to save my vision when others don't have the same opportunity? It sucks.

People will notice. I know that some of the advice I have offered throughout is to help those of us with visual impairment to make our differences less noticeable. I don't do this because I think it is our job to make others around us more comfortable. It is offered because sometimes it is easier to blend in and to not invite questions. A misdirected gaze in one eye, a drooping eyelid, a discolored eye, or a misshapen pupil can be off-putting. From my own experience, I know that an encounter with someone can become more about the undercurrent that occurs because of my bad eye than about the conversation that is taking place. Sometimes people find it unsettling to look directly at me while I'm speaking or on the flip side, they stare too intently at the bad eye trying to figure it out. Or when I see people turning their head to see what they imagine that I might be looking at because my bad eye is drifting, I am at a loss and sometimes have made the point of saying, "My right eye has a mind of its own, just ignore it." And sometimes I say nothing and just continue with the conversation, or, worse still, I find myself looking down so that they don't have to look at my eyes and I don't have to try to guess what they are thinking. To be honest, it's hard for me to really know if it is the bad eye causing the issue and I remind myself that people are mostly concerned with themselves, so someone may be avoiding eye contact because they can't decide which eye to focus on, or maybe it has zero do to with me or my bad eye. Autism, and the million different ways it can present itself, can make direct eye contact too painful for those who have it. And people with social anxiety might also avoid direct eye contact.

One time, when we had a new employee at work, he and I had talked on several occasions before I made a point of telling him that I was visually impaired. "I thought maybe there was something wrong with your eye," he said, "but I didn't want to ask." I gave a quick rundown that the eye was blind, that I do sometimes bang into things on that side, and that it is helpful if he approached me or handed me things on my visual side. Now, this was a really sweet young man who had just graduated from college and was in his first professional job. I know he wanted to say something to make me feel better. "You'll be just fine even with only one eye," he said. "My family had a dog with only three legs and he was just fine." I had to laugh at the comparison. I didn't ask if the dog was gainfully employed and could also drive a car, two activities that I need to complete on a daily basis.

The truth is, people expect symmetry. Human biology seeks it out. It makes people more attractive to others. Should those of us with visual differences try to make our differences less noticeable? I'm not sure if stating the obvious up front makes it better, or does it change the encounter and focus it on the impairment, or does it embarrass the other person, or does it get the eye issue out of the way so the real conversation can take place as intended? Should people with sight-impairment, or those with autism, or those with limb differences, (an issue my ex-husband dealt with daily after losing the better part of his right arm to Ewing's Sarcoma), or people with a hundred other different abilities, push back against human nature, biology, and the ableist world that tells us the secret to success is to look people directly in the eye and offer a firm handshake? I don't have the answers to any of these questions, but it is something that I spend more time thinking about since I lost the vision in my right eye.

Chapter Ten:
The Upshot and the Three Vows to Myself

I'm happy to report that I am ten years out from my eye surgery experiences and I was able to keep the three vows that I made to myself after the very first surgery.

I did my best to be a good mom to my daughters, and both just recently earned their college degrees and are on the path to becoming productive and well-rounded adults. It wasn't always easy, with my eye surgeries and visual issues and their father's poor health. Unfortunately, he passed away recently, maybe not directly from a lifetime of cancer, but most definitely from his kidneys and liver dealing with a lifetime of pain meds and other medications that gave him more years than anyone would have expected. I felt that even though he and I didn't remain married, we did work as a team to do the best we could in raising our daughters. We seemed in some ways lucky, that when I was down after a surgery, he was able to do more and by the same token, during times when his health suffered, I was able to do more. It worked. I miss him and it makes me really sad that he won't get to see the wonderful things our daughters will experience and become as they grow into adulthood.

My second vow to myself was that I refused to let the eye situation become an issue between me and my man. It wasn't always easy to spend time together, especially when I had to use all of my time off from work for surgery and for medical appointments. But we managed and we are still together. Ours is still a long-distance relationship but we talk every day and see each other as often as possible. We are making plans to live closer to each other once we retire. Will we always be together? That's hard for anyone to say, but if we do split up, it won't be the result of the eye issues. Going through it all together let me see that when the chips were down and things were rough, he didn't flinch or waver. Okay, and the fact that he is really smart, handsome, and funny works in his favor too.

What about the vow that I wouldn't let the never-ending eye surgeries take me under financially? That was a tough one because it is common knowledge that medical expenses are one of the leading causes of bankruptcy. I am fortunate that I had insurance, and even high deductible insurance goes a long way when a person is facing a catastrophic illness and huge medical bills.

I will share that most hospitals and even surgery centers are nonprofit entities. I don't make a ton of money working at a library, but prior to these surgeries, I was able to manage alright on my salary. (And I never sought alimony or child support when my ex-husband and I split up, so I was truly squeaking by on my own salary. One of my former bosses thought this was unheard of and said, "Everyone wants to be divorced from you!" I don't think it was a compliment.) But even though I did not consider myself poor, I applied for financial assistance to any and all of the hospitals and surgery centers where I was a patient. It took an afternoon or two to gather up all of the required information, but each time, I was granted at least a small partial write-off of my balances.

I was able to set up monthly payments to everyone involved and my mom insisted on helping me for several months. Because I still had frequent checkups, I made a point of visiting the surgery wing of the building to make payments in-person and to help myself to a delicious mocha latte at the self-service coffee bar in the waiting room. I felt entitled to it and in a small way, it made up for all of the time I spent in the waiting room before a surgery when I could smell the self-serve coffee bar but couldn't have any. Nobody ever chased me away or asked me what I was doing, so I guess it was okay.

This might make it sound like wading through the financial mess created by the surgeries was easy. It wasn't. But I was determined that I wouldn't go under financially, and so I learned how to hustle to make ends meet. I cleaned houses, did yard work, and helped manage rentals, cleaning and painting in between tenants. I sold stuff on eBay. It was exhausting on top of a full time job. Still, even with side gigs, there were weeks where I barely squeaked by. I knew exactly how many packages of chicken or hamburger I had in the freezer and if I was going to have enough food for the number of meals we would need before the next payday. I also knew exactly (most of the time) how many miles to the gallon my car could go and whether or not the tank would be on E before I got paid again. But sometimes, like in everyone's life, unexpected expenses came up, like a car repair, a school skating party, or an order form for a band t-shirt. If it wasn't in my tight budget, I had to get creative. This led me to visit a payday lender on at least one occasion, and even though the interest rate was sky high, I was willing to pay it. It was worth it to stop worrying about how I was going to pay for whatever the unexpected expense was. Another "skill" I learned was how to use a pawnshop. I have a couple of decent pieces of jewelry that I would never sell because they mean too much to me. However, I quickly learned that a decent piece of jewelry was worth $80 at a pawnshop and paying back $90 within the next two weeks didn't seem so bad if it was just enough to scrape by and make up the amount needed to cover a shortfall. When I drive past the payday loan place or the pawnshop now, it's hard to not give a quick prayer of thanks that these were temporary fixes in my life. I feel bad for people who fall into the cycle of payday loans or pawning things when they don't have any light or any hope at the end of the financial tunnel.

So while it may seem at first that I was lucky enough to avoid financial ruin as a result of the surgeries, I have to confess that the experience of working hard and working a lot led me to an almost hopeless place where I threw my arms up in the air regarding my finances in general. I started thinking, "So what if I budget and save when all it takes is one more surgery to wipe out all of my hard work?" I decided that it didn't matter what I did and that I was at the mercy of the situation. This, obviously, was a horrible attitude and it led me to be careless in using credit and credit cards to cover financial obligations. And even though the medical bills were behind me after a few years, it was just in time for some major repairs to my house and for my daughters to start college. I wasn't prepared financially for any of this.

A few years after the surgery saga appeared to be over, my man asked me where I was in terms of my finances, and I couldn't tell him because I didn't know anymore. Several months later, I got up the courage to add it all up and I was shocked at the amount of debt. Living beyond my means by just a few hundred dollars a month or putting textbooks for my daughters' college semesters on a credit card here and there added up. A lot.

I knew about Dave Ramsey and decided I would follow his plan. Thankfully, one of my good friends had just come to terms with the amount of debt she had, and we became accountability partners to encourage each other to get out of debt. She finished paying off her debt a few months before I did. Thirty months after writing out my debt snowball, I made the last credit card/loan/personal loan payment and became completely debt free except for my mortgage. And I will attack that next (once I build up my six-month emergency fund, of course, in case there are any Ramsey fans reading this.) I read an article in *The Guardian* recently in which the author was trying to illustrate that the Ramsey plan might have worked for Dave when he had overleveraged himself buying real estate, but that it wouldn't work for a normal person with normal debt. "Wrong!" Math is math and it works for everyone. The writer also described Dave as, "not unhandsome," which in my understanding of the English language equals handsome. Why the double negative? Obviously, the writer had a serious chip on his shoulder and couldn't toss Dave Ramsey even a small bone of kindness. The truth is, Dave Ramsey, his advice, and his baby steps helped me (and millions of others) get to a much better place financially and I will be forever grateful.

Encouragement. I can't lie to you; you will have some dark days when the surgeries and the sight-impairment and the mountain of medical bills seem like too much and the fear of losing what vision you have left is overwhelming. At one checkup, I sat next to an older lady who had a charming British accent. She told me she was from England but had met an American soldier during WWII and became a war bride, spending most of her adult life in the Indianapolis-area. She told me she was widowed now. She was severely diabetic and had lost the vision in one eye to diabetic retinopathy. The previous year, she had suffered a heart attack and would have died, had it not been for a granddaughter who just happened to stop by her house, found her, and called an ambulance.

Through medical intervention, she survived the heart attack. But now she was almost blind in her good eye and was sure that she would soon be entirely blind. She started crying, "If I knew I was going to be totally blind, I wish I would have died that day on my kitchen floor." I patted her arm and told her not to think like that because I'm sure her family members thought every day they had with her was a gift and surely they would love her and help her even if she became totally blind. At least that is what I said out loud. In my own heart and mind, I totally understood what she was saying, and I couldn't blame her a bit. Yes, I know that people who are totally blind have perfectly ordinary and sometimes extraordinary lives. People with physical, sensory, and other differences find ways to persevere and do what they can to the best of their abilities, but, just like that sweet little old lady, I hope I never have to find out how I would cope with total blindness.

I spent a lot of time thinking about total blindness because the detachment in the bad eye was caused by age and nearsightedness. This meant there was no guarantee that the same thing wouldn't happen in my good eye (which is obviously the same age as the bad eye and just as nearsighted.) It is beyond frightening to think about what would happen and how much my life would change if I were to lose the remaining vision I have. I wondered if I should somehow prepare for this eventuality by learning braille or other coping strategies. With each passing year, this fear has lessened as my surgeon spends more time and attention on the good eye and assessing the health of its retina. And to be honest, I know more now than I used to. If a curtain or shadow or fixed wiggly something were to appear now in the vision in my good eye, I would be on my way to see the specialist as soon as possible. And if the retina in the good eye were to detach, maybe now, at ten years out from my initial surgeries, there would be a new therapy or intervention for the proliferative scarring issue. Maybe now the disease doesn't get to win as often.

To anyone reading this who may be experiencing vision loss or who has a loved one who is experiencing vision loss or another medical crisis, I hope that my experiences might help you. Know that whatever you are experiencing, you are not alone. It may feel like it and sometimes you will feel that no one understands what you are going through or how you struggle to get through the day. It is hard. When a cannonball of light shoots through your vision, try to ignore it and know that you are not alone. When you spill a drink or miss a step or smack into a door frame on your bad side for the hundredth time, just take a deep breath and pray for patience and strength, and a sense of humor.

If you are fortunate, like I was, that your health crisis is life-changing but not life-threatening, challenge yourself to make your own vows. Decide what lines you won't let the illness cross. Say it out loud or put it in writing but decide for yourself what you won't let the illness, injury, or disease take from you. You probably won't know at the time how you will make the vows come to pass, but arming yourself with resolve and recognizing what means the most to you will give you strength as you deal with the challenges and realities of your health crisis and its outcomes. God bless you and good luck to us all!

--the end--

About the Author

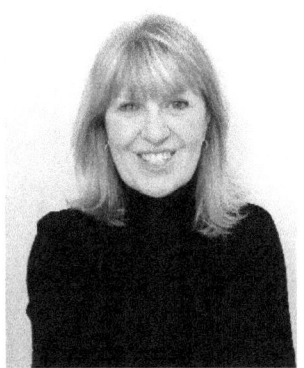

Susan E. Fisher is a resident of Muncie, Indiana. She is the fourth of six siblings in a family of five chatty sisters and one not-so-chatty brother. She is a graduate of Ball State University and has worked in public relations in the nonprofit world for more than 30 years. In this role, she has shared words, pictures, and stories to promote organizations such as United Way, Ball State University, and the Muncie Public Library. She is the mother of two daughters. When she is not working, she enjoys volunteering, attending community events, and spending time with her friends and family.

Susan was diagnosed with a spontaneous detached retina at 47. Despite several surgeries, she lost the vision in one eye. She wrote "Bad Eye" to help others who may be facing eye surgery and vision loss. She hopes her experiences can help others recognize the warning signs of a detached retina and she offers ideas of how to navigate everyday life with single eye vision.

Susan holds a B.S. in journalism, public relations, and marketing from Ball State University.

Credits: Photo by Tommy Garrett Photography
tommygarrett1@gmail.com.

Bad Eye fish illustration by Carly Fisher
carlyannefisher@gmail.com.

www.ingramcontent.com/pod-product-compliance
Lightning Source LLC
Chambersburg PA
CBHW070512220526
45467CB00002B/624